Frequently Asked Questions

all about
omega-3 oils

CLARA FELIX

D1413656

AVERY PUBLISHING GROUP

Garden City Park • New York

The information contained in this book is based upon the research and personal and professional experiences of the author. It is not intended as a substitute for consulting with your physician or other health care provider. Any attempt to diagnose and treat an illness should be done under the direction of a health care professional.

The publisher does not advocate the use of any particular health care protocol, but believes the information in this book should be available to the public. The publisher and author are not responsible for any adverse effects or consequences resulting from the use of any of the suggestions, preparations, or procedures discussed in this book. Should the reader have any questions concerning the appropriateness of any procedure or preparation mentioned, the author and the publisher strongly suggest consulting a professional health care advisor.

Series cover designer: Eric Macaluso
Cover image courtesy of Steven Foster Group, Inc.

Avery Publishing Group, Inc.
120 Old Broadway, Garden City Park, NY 11040
1-800-548-5757 or visit us at www.averypublishing.com

ISBN: 0-89529-889-9

Printed in the United States of America

10   9   8   7   6   5   4   3   2   1

Contents

Introduction

Confused about oils? Can't tell the difference between good and bad fats and oils? You're far from alone. But after reading *All About Omega-3 Oils*, you'll have a clear understanding of the dietary fats that can reduce your risk of heart disease and cancer, ease your aches and pains, and relieve a variety of other conditions. While many fats are not good for health, at least when consumed in excess, the omega-3 oils—sometimes referred to as "fish oils"—are good for health.

Why so much confusion over dietary fats? It all goes back to a big mistake made in medicine some fifty years ago. That's when the experts decided the American public needed a "transfusion" of polyunsaturated oils to stop the growing epidemic of heart attacks. The fundamental error they made was to leave out the special fats you will be reading about here—the omega-3 family of essential fatty acids. America's diet was already too sparse in good fats, but when the few omega-3s that still remained in foods were drowned out by a glut of other polyun-saturated oils, the deficiency hit a danger point.

Now many serious diseases are being reversed or, better yet, avoided when these special fats are restored to their rightful place in the diet. Yet most doctors and dietitians remain in the dark about the role of the omega-3s in health. You may have to be the one to enlighten your doctor. You'll probably want to when you see what happens to your health after you make the simple changes in your diet described in this book.

In the following pages, you'll find out what a fatty acid is, what makes the omega-3s unique, and why so many common annoyances, such as dry skin and achy joints, are improved when these fats are put back into the diet. You'll also learn about the role of the omega-3s in improving disorders such as asthma and allergies, and in preventing serious, life-threatening illnesses such as heart disease, dia-betes, and cancer. In addition, you'll learn why these special fats are often called "brain food," and how they can change your disposition from grumpy to sunny.

The most encouraging aspects of the omega-3 "good" oils are how readily they are accepted by the body and how quickly they begin helping the body's healing and renewal efforts. The omega-3 oils truly are "good guys."

1.

Just What Are the Omega-3s?

Few Americans today have never heard the dietary advice to keep your fat intake down to a maximum of 30 percent of your total daily calories. Books and magazine articles abound with tips for cutting the fat out of your diet, and supermarket shelves sag under the weight of the fat-free and reduced-fat products available to accomplish this goal. But not too many people realize that not all fats are bad and that including some good fats in the diet is essential. This chapter will explain what these good fats are and why they are important for a healthy body and brain.

Q. What are the omega-3 oils?

A. The omega-3 oils belong to a very special group of fats called the essential fatty acids, the key word being "essential." In medical terms, this means that these particular fats are necessary for life and health. There's no way you can stay healthy without them. Back in the 1930s, scientists discovered that of all the fats in plant and animal foods, only two had to be obtained from the diet. The two we humans require are in the omega-3 and omega-6 families of the essential fatty acids. Omitting these fatty acids from the diet can bring on serious health consequences—just as if your diet didn't supply you with enough vitamins or essential minerals.

Q. What do the omega-3 oils do for health?

A. Now that medical researchers have been looking at the omega-3s, the list of impressive benefits has been growing. First of all, the omega-3s reduce the risk of heart disease. The omega-3s are natural blood thinners. They keep the blood fats known as triglycerides down at safe levels, lower blood pressure if it's high, and help the arteries to stay elastic and free of inflammation. In general, the omega-3s are needed for good blood circulation.

Second, as natural anti-inflammatory agents, the omega-3s also help to prevent, or ease the symptoms of, ailments such as asthma, arthritis, menstrual cramps, and migraine headaches.

Third, the retinas of the eyes especially need the omega-3 oils for proper vision. In addition, the omega-3s are needed to prevent damage to and increase circulation in the tiny blood vessels in the eyes, just as they benefit the blood vessels to the heart.

Fourth, when you add the omega-3 oils to your diet, you get "brain food." No kidding. The most polyunsaturated of the omega-3s happen to be a big part of your gray matter. Researchers report that in certain countries where lots of fish is eaten, people have very low rates of depression, as compared to the United States, for example, where little fish is consumed and depression is a big problem.

Fifth, the omega-3s reduce the risk of cancer. You'll learn more about this, and about all of the benefits just mentioned, later in this book.

Q. How can I tell if I need to take supplemental omega-3s?

A. Do you have dry skin? This is the first and most common sign of an omega-3 deficiency. Around each and every cell in the skin is a membrane that normally keeps moisture inside the cell. This membrane is, in effect, a natural moisture barrier for the body. The omega-3 fatty acids form a part of this membrane, thus helping to keep the skin hydrated and soft. If you have dry skin, or any of the health problems mentioned above, the chances are that you've been shortchanging yourself of the omega-3 fatty acids, just like the great majority of Americans.

Q. What exactly is a fatty acid?

A. All fats are made of the same basic elements—carbon, oxygen, and hydrogen. These elements are arranged in molecules called "fatty acids." The fatty part of a fatty-acid molecule consists of carbon atoms linked together in a chain. The acid part consists of hydrogen and oxygen atoms, which are attached to the end of the carbon chain. A chain can consist of anywhere from four to twenty-eight carbon atoms. The fatty acid is classified as short-, medium-, or long-chained according to the length of this chain.

Q. What does "polyunsaturated" mean?

A. In a fatty-acid molecule, the carbon chain itself also carries hydrogen atoms. In saturated fats, the carbon chain has as many hydrogen atoms as possible attached to it—that is, the chain is saturated with hydrogen atoms. In unsaturated fats, the carbon chain has fewer hydrogen atoms attached. It has room for more. Unsaturated fats are either monounsaturated or polyunsaturated. In monounsaturated fats, two hydrogen atoms have dropped off from adjacent carbon atoms in the middle of the chain. At this carbon-to-carbon link where the hydrogen atoms dropped off, a double bond has formed, forming a weak spot and causing the chain to kink. Because kinked chains can't bunch snugly together, fats made of monounsaturated fatty acids are less solid and more apt to be fluid at room temperature. Polyunsaturated fats have had even more hydrogen atoms drop off the chain—from four to twelve more atoms. The fewer hydrogen atoms a chain has, the more kinks it has. And the more kinks a chain has, the more fluid the fat is.

Q. Why are some fats called "omega-3s"?

A. The omega-3s are polyunsaturated, meaning they have two or more double bonds in their chains. The name "omega-3" comes from the carbon atom where the first double bond is located (counting from the fats end of the chain). For the omega-3 oils, the first double bond is always at carbon atom number three. For the omega-6 oils, another family of essential fatty acids, the first double bond is always at carbon atom number six.

Q. What are the main omega-3 fats and oils? Does fish oil supply omega-3s?

A. Alpha-linolenic acid (LNA), eicosapentaenoic acid (EPA), and docosahexgenoic acid (DHA) are the chief omega-3 fatty acids. LNA is eighteen carbon atoms long and very unsaturated, containing three double bonds. LNA is described as "18:3n3," which is shorthand for "eighteen carbon atoms, three double bonds, omega-3 family."

When you digest and absorb fats containing LNA, your enzymes may convert some of the LNA into longer, more highly polyunsaturated omega-3 fatty acids. Eicosapentaenoic acid (EPA) and docosahexaenoic acid (DHA) are the most heavily researched of these. EPA is twenty carbon atoms long and has five double bonds (20:5n3). DHA, the most unsaturated omega-3 of all, is twenty-two carbon atoms long, with six double bonds (22:6n3). You need about ten LNAs before your body can convert one into EPA.

LNA comes mainly from plant foods, with good sources being flaxseeds, flaxseed oil, canola oil (from rape seeds), walnuts, and green leafy vegetables such as purslane. Plant foods rarely contain EPA or DHA, which are found in fish oils. The main exception is fresh (not dried) seaweed. Fortunately, seaweed forms a big part of the diets of island and coastal people worldwide.

Fish and shellfish, on the other hand, usually contain just a little LNA, but lots of EPA and DHA, with fish having more than shellfish because their tissues have more fat, most of it EPA and DHA. Therefore, the oils extracted from fish can be concentrated sources of EPA and DHA. Incidentally, whales, seals, and dolphins also have lots of EPA and DHA even though they're mammals. All sea creatures need these super-unsaturated omega-3s for heat and to keep their tissues elastic and flexible in icy waters. You need more omega-3s in cold weather for the same reason.

Q. If the omega-3s and omega-6s both are required for normal health, why the big fuss about the omega-3s?

A. For forty years, doctors have been telling us how vital polyunsaturated fats are for good health, especially the heart. Back in the 1950s, they began worrying about an increase in a new kind of heart attack, not the usual one related to infections, congenital defects, or just plain old age, but one that struck healthy-looking men in their forties and fifties. Autopsies showed arteries narrowed by fatty plaque, with the main artery to the heart blocked. Sadly, the terms "atherosclerosis" and "coronary artery disease" entered our language.

America's eating patterns had greatly changed since the beginning of the Industrial Revolution. Researchers confirmed that two of these changes—too much saturated fat, from meat, and too little polyunsaturated fat—were bad for the heart. In the late 1950s, doctors began to urge people to increase their intake of polyunsaturated fatty acids. They forgot about the omega-3s, however. The food industry responded with tankfuls of polyunsaturated oils, for both commercial and household use. The country was soon awash in corn, safflower, peanut, sunflower, and cottonseed oils, all full of omega-6, but with little or no omega-3.

The oversight was understandable. In those days, far less was known about the essential fatty acids than, say, vitamins, which were discovered decades earlier. Not only were scientists learning how complex fatty acids are, but the technology to analyze and measure them in human tissues was still in its infancy. It was easy for researchers to dismiss the earlier studies about omega-3 and focus on omega-6, which was going "to save the heart."

Luckily, in the 1970s, evidence emerged about how remarkably free of heart disease the Inuits (Eskimos) in Greenland were, even though they ate a lot of fat. It turned out the fat was full of the long-overlooked omega-3s, from the fish and sea mammals that composed their diet. The news fueled a great burst of new studies. Eventually, those studies led to the current awareness that humans have all kinds of problems—from bad complexions, arthritis, immune disorders, and depression, all the way to deadly heart attacks—because we don't get enough omega-3.

Essential Fatty Acids Made Simple

Both families of essential fatty acids are necessary for health. However, the modern diet contains too much of the omega-6 fatty acids compared to the omega-3 fatty acids.

OMEGA-6 FATTY-ACIDS FAMILY	OMEGA-3 FATTY-ACIDS FAMILY
Linoleic acid (LA) (found in vegetable oils)	Alpha-linolenic acid (LNA) (found in dark green vegetables)
Converted in the body to:	*Converted in the body to:*
Gamma-linolenic acid (GLA) (also found in evening primrose and borage oils) *and*	Eicosapentaenoic acid (EPA) (also found in fish oils) *and*
Dihomogammalinolenic acid (DGLA) *and*	Docosahexaenoic acid (DHA) (also found in fish oils)
Arachidonic acid (AA)	

Q. My whole life I have been told that I'm supposed to skip butter and saturated fats, and instead get plenty of polyunsaturated fats. What's wrong with this?

A. One of the toughest tasks that the medical and nutrition policy-setters have been facing is acknowledging that their big push for polyunsaturated fats has backfired. By constantly rhapsodizing about the heart-saving value of the omega-6 oils and margarines, and ignoring the need for the omega-3s, the experts have been encouraging a daily consumption of anywhere from ten to thirty times more omega-6 than omega-3 fatty acids. The scores are in now, and they tell us that this unnatural ratio is making people *more* sick.

High levels of the omega-6 oils without the restraining effects of the omega-3s actually promotes the diseases that are supposed to be prevented. Yes, this includes heart disease, allergies, asthma, autoimmune diseases, obesity, diabetes, depression—even cancer. An important 1997 study from Japan details how all of these diseases began to rise for the first time in Japan's history only after its people began consuming more of the omega-6 oils in their newly "westernized" diet.

Many concerned scientists now are convinced that good health depends on rebalancing our omega intake to no more than three times more omega-6 than omega-3 fatty acids, and to as low as one-to-one for recovery purposes. To put this in perspective, our hunter and gatherer ancestors consumed about equal amounts of omega-6 and omega-3 oils, and this ratio appears to be the ideal for our bodies.

Q. Why aren't we getting enough omega-3s in our food?

A. Some of the best food sources of the omega-3s have gone "out of fashion," even though they used to be diet mainstays. Fish is a good example. In the early days, before food and water were transported by trains, trucks, planes, and pipelines, people always settled near a lake, river, or stream. This assured them not only of water and transportation, but of dependable sources of protein—fish and shellfish. Of all edibles, fish and shellfish are the undisputed omega-3 champions.

The early American settlers also used to depend on wild game for protein. In addition to being high in protein, wild game is also a good source of the omega-3s. Today, we rely on domestically raised beef, which provides almost no omega-3s.

Walnuts and butternuts, good omega-3 sources, used to be staples in American kitchens. Nowadays, people substitute nuts like cashews and peanuts, which have little omega-3s.

Historically, since early Greek and Roman times, flaxseeds and their oil were valued in many parts of the world, but were replaced after World War II with oils that offer little or no omega-3s. There's a big push now to bring flaxseeds back, because flaxseeds and the oil pressed from them provide more omega-3s than almost any other edible seed and oil.

Purslane, a low-growing plant with small fleshy leaves, is enjoyed as a salad green or as a cooked or pickled vegetable in many countries. However, it's scorned as a weed here, even though in earlier times Native Americans cherished purslane as both a food and a medicine. There is something to be said for folk wisdom because, in 1986, Artemis P. Simopoulos, M.D., and her research group discovered purslane to be the highest in omega-3s of any known green leafy vegetable. They also learned that it's super-high in vitamins C and E.

Q. Why is it so easy to get too much of the omega-6 fatty acids?

A. Except in fish and shellfish, the omega-6s are much more available than the omega-3s. For example, everyday sources that take care of your omega-6 requirements include cereal, whole-grain bread, nuts, sunflower seeds, peanuts, beans, eggs, poultry, and pork. Additional oil may not be needed at all.

Whether in the home or the commercial food-processing plant, the lavish use of omega-6 oils, margarine, and mayonnaise for salads, sandwich dressings, baked goods, fried foods, and more is strictly a twentieth-century phenomenon. Before, oil was consumed frugally, since the typical oils such as flaxseed and olive had to be extracted using hand-run presses and were available only seasonally. Animal fats from poultry and pork were staples in most households.

Since the ratio of the two fatty-acid families is all-important, the more omega-6s you consume, the more omega-3s you need. If you don't take in enough omega-3s, a high omega-6 intake spells trouble.

Q. If I cut out most oils and margarine, how can I get enough omega-6s, since they're essential, too?

A. If you eat a reasonably healthy diet, you seldom need extra omega-6 from oils and other supplemental sources. Most of the popular nuts, seeds, and whole grains, and the breads and cereals made with them, supply little omega-3s, but ample omega-6 fatty acids. Chicken, turkey, lamb, and especially pork have hardly any omega-3s, but fair amounts of omega-6s. Although soybeans and their products including tofu, miso, and tempeh are sources of omega-3s, they contain about ten times more omega-6s. Walnuts supply more omega-3s than almost any other nut, but their omega-6 content is more than four times higher. Even flaxseed oil is 15 percent omega-6 (but 55 percent omega-3). Do you see how using lots of omega-6 oils, mayonnaise, and salad dressings can easily upset your fatty-acid balance?

Q. What are trans-fatty acids?

A. Trans-fatty acids are products of today's high-tech treatment of food oils. The more polyunsaturated (liquid) a fat is, the quicker it can become rancid. Hydrogenation of oils, which uses heat and a metal catalyst to force hydrogen atoms back onto the carbon atoms in the fatty-acid chains, was invented in the early 1900s to remedy this. What it produces, though, is a hardened, solid fat that has a long shelf life, but zero essential fatty acids.

A variation of this original treatment, called "light hydrogenation" or "partial hydrogenation," is used today on many oils and most margarines because it doesn't produce a hard fat. Unfortunately, it transforms the targeted omega-6 and omega-3 fatty acids in the oils into unnatural "funny fats" that no longer can do what real essential fatty acids do when consumed except to provide calories. These "funny fats" are the trans-fatty acids. They are found not only in oils and margarine, but in the hundreds of commercial products prepared with these fats.

Trans-fatty acids are sneaky because they resemble true essential fatty acids enough so that your cell membranes accept them eagerly. Once they become part of your tissues, however, they can't do what the omega-6 and omega-3 fatty acids do. The more trans-fatty acids you eat, the bigger your omega-3 deficit becomes.

When the food industry was pressured into using heart-healthy polyunsaturated oils instead of animal fats and tropical fats such as coconut oil, the trans-fatty-acid content of commercial foods shot sky-high. What the crafty commercial food industry had done was to switch to partially hydrogenated oils in order to get the crispy, flaky textures in their products that animal fats and coconut oil used to provide. Even crackers for babies contain partially hydrogenated fat. Health food stores are your best bet for finding packaged goods made with butter, coconut oil, or nonhydrogenated vegetable oil, preferably canola.

Q. Okay, I'll accept that the omega-3s are essential, but why are they so important? What proof is there that they're missing from the diet?

A. Not all doctors thought it was a good idea to ignore the omega-3s. One such doctor was Edward N. Siguel, M.D., Ph.D. Using a new method that he developed to measure the fatty acids in human tissues, he analyzed blood plasma from five hundred "healthy" men and women. The majority proved to have very low levels of the omega-3s and a big imbalance between the omega-3s and omega-6s.

Donald O. Rudin, M.D., was director of molecular biology research at a major psychiatric institute when he determined that the dietary availability of the omega-3 fatty acids had declined to less than 20 percent of the level it had been in traditional American diets. This convinced him that an omega-3 deficiency could be the "missing link" in the rise of such ailments as heart disease, arthritis, obesity, depression, and schizophrenia. In the early 1980s, he set up an informal pilot study with forty-four volunteers, twelve of whom had serious mental illness. All had physical problems that didn't respond to any treatment.

The volunteers took individualized doses of flaxseed oil or fish oil three times a day, along with vitamins E and B. They ate their usual diets, continued their regular medical treatments, and were counseled to avoid using omega-6 oils and margarine.

The results were gratifying beyond expectations. Over a one- to two-year period, the mentally normal subjects experienced improvements in longstanding problems such as arthritis, bursitis, glaucoma, high blood pressure, angina (chest pains upon exertion), tension headaches, irritable bowel syndrome, dry skin, and dermatitis. They also had an increased sense of well-being.

Of the twelve mental patients, at least seven had a reduction in psychotic thinking, along with an improved sense of well-being. Their mental and emotional progress paralleled the improvements in their physical problems including irritable bowel syndrome, arthritis, tinnitus (noises in the head), and very dry skin.

Q. How can a single nutrient such as omega-3 have an effect on so many different ailments?

A. We shouldn't be too surprised. After all, it was one tiny vitamin, niacin, that single-handedly cleared up the "three Ds" of pellagra—diarrhea, dermatitis, and dementia. Some experts added a fourth D, for "death," when terrible pellagra epidemics swept through the South in the early 1900s. An estimated ten thousand people succumbed to the disease in 1915, and another seven thousand died from it as late as 1929. Thousands more ended up in mental institutions. Most of the victims were poor, often subsisting on refined cornmeal, corn grits, lard, and white-flour biscuits. Many authorities were sure pellagra was an infectious disease, but in 1937, very sick patients who were given the experimental B vitamin niacin had "miraculous" recoveries, even from psychosis.

In the late 1960s, scientists determined that prostaglandins, hormone-like compounds that are among the most potent biological substances known, are made in the body solely from omega-3 and omega-6 fatty acids. Both families of essential fatty acids are needed in the diet to form this newly discovered body-wide regulatory system. Prostaglandins and related molecules made from omega-3 and omega-6 fatty acids are grouped together under the term "eicosanoids." Eicosanoids have been proven to be as powerful as such hormones as insulin, secreted by the pancreas. Insulin, however, circulates in the blood, while eicosanoids exert their influence locally in the cells and tissues in which they are made. Science finally discovered one big reason why the essential fatty acids are essential—the eicosanoids your body makes from them have a finger in every pie because they affect every organ system.

Q. What eventually convinced medical researchers that both omega-6s and omega-3s are needed in the diet?

A. Prostaglandins (or eicosanoids) can have good and bad effects. Bad effects can arise when we produce an excess of certain eicosanoids. The most potentially harmful ones are made in our cells from arachidonic acid (AA), an omega-6. Because there was resistance in the medical world to accepting any need for the omega-3s, it was difficult for the small group of researchers who knew better to get their views published in the medical journals.

The Greenland Eskimo discovery changed all that. Funding became available for worldwide studies on the omega-3s and the heart. The medical world waited with great excitement for the results, which quickly appeared in the prestigious journals. That's how it learned that the omega-3s put the brakes on overproduction of the omega-6 eicosa-noids, which are responsible for the mischief in the arteries.

Nature apparently meant for us to get both fami-lies of fatty acids from our foods. *Balance*—this is what it is all about—and that's what is missing from most Americans' diets.

2.

Heart Disease and Cancer

In this chapter, we will take a look at two health matters that are closely tied to the omega oils. One is atherosclerosis, the most thoroughly researched of the omega-related conditions. The other is cancer, also a problem of our modern age related to omega deficiency.

Q. Can the omega-3 fatty acids really help to prevent heart attacks and strokes?

A. Yes, through a number of mechanisms. For one, the omega-3 oils prevent unneeded blood clots from forming by keeping in check an eicosanoid known as thromboxane, made from the omega-6 fatty acid AA. Clotting initiated by normal levels of thromboxane is necessary to keep you from bleeding to death from injury, but abnormal clotting from too much thromboxane is dangerous. Blood clots where they're not needed can shut off circulation to any part of the body. If a clot (thrombus) keeps enough blood from getting to the brain or heart, it can trigger a stroke or heart attack. Dr. Edward N. Siguel has suggested that higher blood levels of the omega-3 fatty acid EPA may serve as an alternative to aspirin for reducing clotting and preventing heart disease, with practically no side effects.

The omega-3s also have the unique ability to reduce high levels of triglycerides, a fat in the blood. According to omega-3 researcher William Harris, Ph.D., professor of medicine at the University of Missouri, Kansas City, an elevated triglyceride level now is recognized as an important risk factor for heart disease.

The omega-3s join with the omega-6s in your system to form special lipids, or fats, that compose the structural membranes of every single cell in your body. These membranes are like the walls of a house. So, in addition to creating eicosanoids, the omega-3 and omega-6 oils help to control all the substances that go in and out of your cells, acting, in effect, like doorways. The omega-3s increase the flexibility of the red-blood-cell membranes, enabling these blood cells to swim more freely through the bends and turns of the tiny capillaries. They actually make your blood less sludgy and more fluid. This not only improves circulation everywhere in the body, including the brain, but makes it easier for the heart to do its job of continuous pumping.

Q. Do the omega-3s affect the heart and arteries directly?

A. High blood pressure can lead to both a stroke and a heart attack. One factor is too much of that same omega-6 eicosanoid, thromboxane. Thromboxane is a potent constrictor of your arteries. The omega-3s help to normalize high blood pressure by—you guessed it—stopping overproduction of thromboxane and by allowing the blood vessels to stretch out and relax.

The *New England Journal of Medicine* reported recently that hardened and narrowed arteries (atherosclerosis) associated with stroke and heart attack can be caused by chronic inflammation in blood-vessel walls. This inflammation starts much like the redness and swelling when a cut in your finger becomes infected, but, according to researchers, the overactive immune-system cells in the blood vessels may keep the inflammation going, turning a defense measure into a destructive one. It has even been suggested that this kind of chronic inflammation is a more fundamental cause of atherosclerosis than are high cholesterol or high blood pressure. So, by reining in the omega-6 eicosanoids before they can set off a chain reaction leading to inflammation in the arteries, the omega-3s play still another role in preventing heart disease.

The omega-3s also help your heartbeat. Heart attacks aren't always deadly, but they can become lethal if your heart responds by going into wildly uncontrolled arrhythmic quivering known as fibrillation, keeping the blood from reaching vital organs including the brain. Omega-3 fatty acids from fish oils specifically help to prevent arrythmia. They also slow down a too-fast heartbeat by actually decreasing the electrical excitability of the heart-muscle cells.

Q. Can the omega-3s help people who already have blood-vessel problems?

A. Artemis P. Simopoulos, M.D., suggests that the omega-3 fatty acids can even help people with advanced coronary artery disease. Proof comes from two famous studies, the "DART" trial in England and the Lyon Diet Heart Study in France. In both of these large trials, men who were recovering from heart attacks were placed on one of two diets. Half of the men consumed the diet recommended by heart specialists and the American Heart Association, the so-called "prudent" diet, which was high in omega-6 and low in omega-3 oils. The other half of the men consumed a high-omega-3 diet. Many more patients survived on the omega-3 regimen—so much so that after two years, Dr. Simopoulos reports, the French study was abruptly ended for ethical reasons because the new diet was proving so superior.

In Dr. Donald O. Rudin's informal pilot study, two patients who suffered angina pectoris (pain in the chest resulting from poor blood supply to the heart upon exertion) "reported a complete disappearance of pain within several months after starting the flaxseed-oil regimen," Dr. Rudin writes. A circulatory problem known as intermittent claudication hampered one volunteer's ability to walk even short distances without getting crippling leg pains. Flaxseed oil brought relief within a few months.

"Another circulatory problem, Raynaud's disease—in which blood vessels in the hands and feet constrict abnormally, causing icy coldness—was greatly diminished in two patients," Rudin writes.

Q. I heard that the omega-3s can prevent cancer. Is this true?

A. The experts generally agree that a vigorous immune system is your best defense against cancer.

But like the other systems in your body, the immune system has to be nourished. Even when your diet provides all the essentials, if the balance of omega-3 to omega-6 oils is off, your immune defenses won't be up to par. According to Dr. Simopoulos, different fats affect tumor growth in different ways. Generally, fats high in omega-6 fatty acids encourage tumor growth, while fats high in omega-3 fatty acids block tumor growth.

A very new finding is that the omega-3 fatty acids can actually create special "roadblocks" in the body, making it harder for cancer cells to migrate from a primary tumor and start new colonies. Cancers that spread (metastasize) are the real killers.

In South Africa, a group of researchers compared the rate of colon cancer in the people living in a small fishing village with the rate in a group of similar people living in urban Cape Town. They found that the city dwellers had six times more colon cancer than the villagers. At first they couldn't understand this. The city dwellers seemed to be eating double the fruits and vegetables as the villagers, for example, and their diet contained more of the nutrients known to protect against colon cancer—fiber, calcium, and antioxidants. Lab tests provided the reason, however—the villagers had three times more omega-3 fatty acids in their blood because of the high amount of fish in their diet and considerably less omega-6 fatty acids, with the ratio between omega-6 and omega-3 being much healthier.

Q. What about flaxseeds? How do they fight cancer?

A. It appears that in the South African study, discussed above, the omega-3s in fish were the key. Flaxseeds, however, provide a unique protective substance in addition to omega-3 fatty acids. Not only do these little brown seeds contain cancer-fighting LNA, the building block of other omega-3 fatty acids, they also supply a special fiber called lignan. In your body, lignan turns into compounds called mammalian lignans, which show big promise as deterrents to breast, colon, and prostate cancers. In lab experiments using flaxseeds, lignans have blocked the formation of new tumors, while LNA has slowed the growth of existing ones. The combination has shrunk breast tumors in rats by more than half.

There's a special bonus you get from flaxseeds—they help your body to produce from seventy-five to eight hundred times more of these protective mammalian lignans than it would if you ate any of the other best sources, such as beans and bran.

French researchers monitoring 120 breast-cancer patients over a three-year period learned that the women who had high levels of LNA in the tissues surrounding their breasts were far better able to keep their cancers from spreading to other parts of their bodies. Breast cancer was five times more likely to metastasize in women with low levels of LNA.

Now that we have the science to explain flax-seeds' benefits, it's easy to see why the seeds and their oil have been valued by human societies for thousands of years. Dr. Simopoulos, who grew up in Greece, notes that even Pliny refered to Greek flaxseed bread.

3.

Brain Function

The omega fatty acids have been shown to play a prominent role in mental health. A number of mental disorders, including depression and schizophrenia, may very well be manifestations of an omega-3 deficiency. In this chapter, we'll take a look at some of the common mental disorders and their connections to the omega-3 and omega-6 oils.

Q. Why are the omega-3s often called "brain food"?

A. Your brain is composed mostly of fats called lipids, including cholesterol and monounsaturated and polyunsaturated fats. While your body can make cholesterol and most brain lipids from scratch, it depends on foods containing the omega-6 and omega-3 fatty acids to assemble the polyunsaturates. The omega-6 fatty acid AA and the omega-3 fatty acid DHA are the most abundant polyunsaturated fats in your brain, with DHA predominating.

When you were a fetus in the womb, the placenta supplied you with AA and DHA derived from your mother's diet, or from her tissues if her diet didn't have enough. If a pregnant woman supplies her fetus with omega-6s but not enough omega-3s, nature tries to compensate by transforming omega-6s into longer-chained, more polyunsaturated fats resembling DHA. The resemblance may fall short in performance, however. An experiment demonstrated the difference—juvenile rats, born to dams that had been deprived of omega-3s, developed brains full of omega-6 DHA-substitutes. Compared with rats born to omega-3-nourished dams, the deprived juveniles showed behavioral abnormalities and didn't do nearly as well in maze tests.

Incidentally, the more fish and other omega-3 foods a pregnant woman includes in her daily diet, the more DHA she provides her unborn baby, and the lower the chance that either she or the baby will be deprived. The same holds true when the infant arrives and starts to breast-feed. In 1997, the American Academy of Pediatrics issued wise new guidelines urging mothers to breast-feed for at least a year—six months longer than previously advised.

Q. If a mother can't or won't breast-feed, how can her baby get DHA?

A. As of this writing, American manufacturers of baby formula are not yet required to add DHA to their products. European, Japanese, and Korean manufacturers several years ago started adding DHA and AA to formulas for premature infants. Now they're beginning to add these brain-building fatty acids to formulas for full-term infants. The hope is that the formula makers in the United States will catch up soon.

In the old days, mothers gave babies a few drops of cod-liver oil a day. Nowadays, special DHA made from either fish oil or vegetarian marine algae is available. A month-old baby from a well-nourished mother gets about 175 milligrams of DHA a day from breast milk, so that might be used as a dosage guide.

Q. How does a mother's alcohol intake affect the level of omega-3s in her unborn baby?

A. Alcohol robs the fetus, and the mother, of DHA. Although the brain normally holds on tenaciously to DHA, it suffers a drop in its DHA content when alcohol is consumed. Alcohol intake does the same thing in the retina of the eye, which needs DHA to convert incoming images into swift electrical signals to be sent to the brain. These findings are based on animal experiments, but human babies born with fetal alcohol syndrome—severe physical abnormalities and mental retardation—are living witnesses to the damage a human mother's drinking can inflict.

British researchers Graham Burdge and Anthony Postle saw comparable defects in newborn guinea pigs that had been exposed to alcohol as fetuses. But when they fed tuna oil enriched with DHA to pregnant guinea pigs throughout gestation along with the alcohol, the abnormalities in the newborn pups were less severe. They're in agreement with Robert Pawlosky and Norman Salem, Jr. from the National Institute on Alcoholism and Alcohol Abuse of the National Institutes of Health (NIH), who say that a pregnant woman who drinks should be given omega-3 supplements in the hope of lessening the damage to her system and to that of her unborn baby.

Q. What about aging and the omega-3s?

A. At the other end of the lifeline, we've got evidence that one of the kindest things you can do for your brain is to keep your DHA reservoirs filled. Dr. Ernst Schaefer of Tufts University measured the DHA in the plasma of more than a thousand healthy sixty-five-year-olds. In the follow-up nine years later, he learned that the folks who had had the lowest DHA levels at the beginning of the study had had a 160-percent greater chance of becoming senile. In the Netherlands, researchers examining the diets of nine hundred elderly men learned that the men who consumed the most omega-6 linoleic acid (LA) were the most likely to suffer from senile dementia. The best mental function belonged to the old men who ate the most fish.

Alzheimer's disease has an inflammatory component to it, as shown by autopsy. Pro-inflammatory elements are seen to be concentrated in the parts of the brain where the most damage from the disease took place. Again, to protect yourself from harm to your priceless thinking machine, you should make sure that your diet is full of naturally anti-inflammatory omega-3 foods and oils. Along with these, consume antioxidant nutrients, such as vitamins A, E, and C, the mineral selenium, and natural carotenoids, polyphenols, and bioflavonoids from foods and supplements, to protect your brain tissues from oxidative damage.

Q. What evidence is there that fatty-acid imbalances can affect your outlook on life?

A. As noted earlier, nearly all of Dr. Rudin's forty-four patients reported feeling calmer and less anxious by the end of his one- to two-year informal pilot study in the early 1980s. Dr. Rudin was one of the first American physicians to treat patients by having them add omega-3 oils to their diets while eliminating or cutting back on omega-6 oils and margarines.

Since then, researchers have noted that populations which use fish as a main protein source have very low rates of major depression. Joseph R. Hibbeln and Norman Salem, Jr. of the NIH note that North American and European populations have a rate of depression ten times greater than that of the people of Taiwan. Fish consumption is high and the rate of depression is low also in Japan and Hong Kong. Many leading scientists agree that the alarming step-up in major depression here may have some roots in the overconsumption of omega-6 oils, coupled with skimpy omega-3 intake. In 1996, an Australian medical group examined the fatty-acid levels in twenty patients suffering from depression and found that the more severe a patient's depressive symptoms were, the higher was the ratio of omega-6 AA to omega-3 EPA in the blood. EPA, supplied along with DHA in fish oil, plays a big role in keeping AA-generated eicosanoids from running amuck.

Postpartum depression, it's suggested, may be

linked to very low DHA in the mother if her reserves are being robbed to nurture the baby because of a low omega-3 intake during pregnancy. And, believe it or not, the severe depression that commonly accompanies alcoholism may also have an omega-3 connection, since alcohol depletes the brain of its stores of DHA.

Q. Is there a fatty-acid connection to attention deficit hyperactivity disorder (ADHD)?

A. ADHD has rapidly grown to become the most common of all the childhood behavior problems. Children with ADHD tend to drive their parents and teachers to distraction because they are chronically inattentive, impulsive, and hyperactive. The accepted treatment of today is stimulant drugs such as Ritalin, but, according to Dr. Simopoulos, physicians may one day prescribe fish for dinner instead, since a link was found between fatty acids and ADHD when it was discovered that boys with ADHD have significantly lower levels of both EPA and DHA than boys without the disorder.

DHA is necessary for the normal functioning of the eyes and the brain's cerebral cortex, the part of the brain that handles the higher functions such as reasoning and memory. Also, ADHD affects many more boys than girls. It so happens that boys require more omega-3, both before and after birth.

ADHD children also tend to have more allergies, eczema, asthma, headaches, stomachaches, ear infections, and dry skin than non-ADHD youngsters do. Dr. Rudin considers these complaints to be part of what he calls the "modernization-disease syndrome," arising from malnutrition stemming from an omega-3 deficiency. Is it only a coincidence that the number of ADHD children in the United States is rising at the same time the trans-fatty-acid content of packaged foods and fast foods is rapidly increasing? Bakery goods, french fries, chips, and other snacks that children love are now full of trans-fatty acids made from partially hydrogenated oils. As these "funny fats" continue to displace the already inadequate omega-3s in children's tissues, the result is a weakening of vital activities that only the omega-3s can reverse.

Q. What about schizophrenia and the omega-3s?

A. Schizophrenia is a mental illness that usually shows up in adolescence or early adulthood. It's often characterized by delusions and hallucinations. Tests show that schizophrenics typically have lowered amounts of the omega-6 and omega-3 fatty acids in their red-blood-cell phospholipids. Phospholipid molecules containing the polyunsaturates form all the cellular membranes, including those of the brain, and one theory is that schizophrenics have a genetic defect that causes their membrane phospholipids to break down at an abnormally high rate. Psychiatrist Malcolm Peet of Sheffield, England, reports that supplementing patients with 10 gm a day of concentrated fish oil "led to significant improvement in schizophrenic symptoms." In a further trial, omega-3 EPA brought about better results than either DHA or a placebo. Dr. Peet says it's not yet clear why EPA is effective while DHA is not. One possibility is that EPA inhibits the enzyme that causes the excessive loss of the membrane phospholipids, but DHA doesn't.

The most remarkable recovery in Dr. Rudin's study was experienced by a twenty-six-year-old woman who had been hospitalized repeatedly since the age of sixteen, when she had first become schizophrenic. Her parents had gotten every possible treatment for her, but nothing had worked for long. Incredibly, the girl responded within thirty minutes to the 2 tbsp of flaxseed oil plus a vitamin-E supplement that Dr. Rudin had recommended. She continued the flaxseed oil and a high-omega-3 diet for several years, went to college, and eventually became a registered nurse in a psychiatric hospital.

Your body's enzymes can convert the LNA you get from dietary flaxseed oil into EPA. Dr. Rudin's forty-four volunteers, who ate a standard American diet, proved to be deficient in the omega-3s. More research is needed, but an intriguing new theory is that EPA stops the excessive destruction of the vital phospholipids.

Q. Is there a connection between anger and irritability, and fatty-acid levels?

A. Hostility and aggression may be aggravated by today's high-omega-6 and low-omega-3 diet. For instance, violent behavior among younger Japanese has taken a sharp upturn, and maybe it's not just the influence of television and movies. Younger people, according to Dr. Harumi Okuyama, are the biggest consumers of the commercial foods that are soaked in high-omega-6 LA and eat less seafood than older Japanese. A double-blind test in which university students were monitored for hostile acts and aggressive behavior against others during a school year, showed only normal behavior by the students who were supplemented with DHA. The control group, which received placebos with no DHA, showed a big rise in aggression and hostility.

Hostility also can kill people by a different route. Hostile folks themselves get more heart attacks. So do depressed persons. Sure, if you're angry or depressed most of the time, your stress hormones are going full blast, which takes a toll on all bodily systems. Also, you're probably not taking care of your health in other ways. But researchers Hibbeln and Salem offer a theory: All three conditions—hostility, depression, and heart disease—may stem from an underlying omega-3 fatty-acid deficiency.

4.

Dry Skin, Diabetes, Arthritis, and More

Do you have bad skin? Are you carrying around a few extra pounds? Are premenstrual syndrome and menstrual cramps regular monthly visitors? Before you run to your doctor or request a referral to a specialist, give the omega-3s a try. The omega-3 oils play a role in every cell of your body, and you just might find that bringing your omega levels back into balance will return that sparkle to your eye and help you stand a little straighter.

Q. My skin is dry and flaky. Can the omega-3 fish oils help?

A. Not just the fish oils—flaxseed oil can help, too. Within a matter of months, Dr. Rudin's pilot-study subjects noticed that the sore, dry, fissured skin on their hands had gotten softer and smoother, their shins had lost their scaly skin flakes, and their cracked, sore heels had healed. The permanent "goose bumps," known as phrynoderma or follicular keratosis, disappeared from their upper arms, thighs, and buttocks. Many found relief from their nonstop dandruff. Eczema, a synonym for dermatitis, which means "inflammation of the skin," was relieved in more than half of the study volunteers who had it. Flaxseed oil worked this "magic" in most of the subjects, but in those whose skin wasn't responding, switching to fish oils usually got results.

Many skin disorders, including psoriasis, have an inflammatory component. Usually, that means the omega-6 eicosanoids are stirring up mischief. Yes, these troublemakers can set off persistent inflammation in the skin even if there's no infection—just the way they've been known to do in blood vessels, joints, and muscles. The omega-3s tend to restrain them by competing for the same enzymes that the omega-6s use to turn into eicosanoids. Japanese doctors saw improvement of red, scaling skin lesions in six out of seven psoriasis patients who took 3.6 gm daily of EPA (from fish oil). At the same time, tests showed a big drop in the omega-6 eicosanoids responsible for inflammation.

Q. Will the omega-3 oils make me fatter? I seem to gain weight from just looking at food.

A. The omega-3 oils won't make you fatter, and they may even help you to lose weight. More than half of all Americans today are overweight, a matter of concern because overweight and obesity often go hand-in-hand with serious health matters such as adult-onset diabetes. Dr. Rudin says obesity "is just one more disease of modernization, caused by a deficiency of essential fatty acids and other vital nutrients, combined with a surplus of antinutrients." The missing fatty acids are the omega-3s, of course, and the "antinutrients" run the gamut from sugar and alcohol all the way to trans-fatty acids.

This combination of nutrient deficiency and antinutrient surplus can undermine the efficiency of your body's appetite-controlling mechanisms. As an example, the satiety center in your brain may not send the right signals, so your appetite stays high long after you've satisfied your body's true needs. An omega-3 deficiency affects your body's heat-controlling, calorie-burning system, too. "As a result," Dr. Rudin writes, "you take in more calories than you burn off."

You'll be comforted to know the omega-3 oils are

the last to be deposited as body fat. As a matter of fact, your body will burn LNA for heat much faster than it will saturated fats like stearic acid and twice as fast as LA.

That's really not surprising because the omega-3 oils are cold-climate fats. They're needed by all aquatic creatures—the colder the water, the more omega-3s are needed in the tissues. The omega-3s also help to regulate fat distribution and fur growth in land animals to protect against cold weather. Most important for you, the omega-3s play a role in how many calories from food are dissipated as heat to warm your body, rather than burned as energy or stored as fat.

Q. It seems that so many people I know are developing diabetes as they get older. Is there a fatty-acid connection?

A. Adult-onset diabetes (diabetes mellitus type II) is definitely on the rise. People who are seriously overweight are especially vulnerable. For one thing, in obesity, the tissues become "insulin resistant"— that is, the muscle cells don't respond properly when told by insulin, the hormone secreted by the pancreas, to take in sugar (glucose) and amino acids from the blood. As a result, the blood-glucose level stays too high, which signals the pancreas to send out even more insulin. Super amounts of insulin are secreted before the muscle cells finally respond, resulting in chronically high blood levels of insulin—not a healthy situation.

Obesity, elevated insulin levels, and insulin resistance can be forerunners to adult-onset diabetes. Adult-onset is different from juvenile diabetes, in which the pancreas stops producing enough insulin. The same problems that generate adult-onset diabetes can also cause high blood pressure, high levels of blood fats, and low levels of high-density lipoprotein (HDL, or good cholesterol). The combination is practically a blueprint for coronary-artery disease.

While a juvenile-onset diabetic usually is underweight and an adult-onset diabetic is overweight, both can suffer from serious muscle wasting because not enough amino acids, the building blocks of protein, get into their muscle tissues. Australian researchers found that rats became insulin resistant on a high-saturated-fat diet. However, when enough omega-3 fatty acids were added to the animals' rations, DHA (the most polyunsaturated fat of all) began to show up in cell membranes in muscle. At that point, the rats' muscle cells regained sensitivity to insulin. Apparently, if cell membranes contain enough DHA, they become elastic and fluid, and, in turn, receptive to insulin. Now we have studies showing that people whose muscle cells have lots of omega-6 but little omega-3 (especially DHA) tend to be insulin resistant, too. They also are more likely to be obese. We've come full circle here.

Q. Some of my friends use omega-3 fish oils to ease arthritic aches and pains. Is there scientific evidence to back this up?

A. The more scientists explore the ways in which eicosanoids control our cellular life, the easier it is to understand why things go wrong in the body. For one thing, persistent inflammation is proving to be the "tie that binds" many different ailments. To explain, overconsumption of the omega-6 fatty acids coupled with underconsumption of the omega-3s is a major trigger for stubborn inflammations that keep simmering even when there's no infection that set them off. Osteoarthritis, the most common form of arthritis, often has an inflammatory component, just as heart disease does. If your diet doesn't cover your omega-3 needs, it won't have the "muscle" needed to knock out the pain- and inflammation-causing omega-6 eicosanoids.

More double-blind experiments need to be done using omega-3 supplements for osteoarthritis, but in his pilot study, Dr. Rudin observed improvement or actual healing over a one- to two-year period in the majority of volunteers who suffered from chronic arthritis or bursitis. Anecdotal evidence may not cut the mustard in medical circles, but lots of it keeps accumulating about how milled flaxseed, flaxseed oil, and fish oil ease osteoarthritis pain and disability when added to the diets of humans as well as pet dogs and cats. Luckily, a number of scientific experiments with laboratory mice back up these results.

Rheumatoid arthritis is a more serious kind of arthritis, involving inflammation that can destroy joint tissues. In sixteen major double-blind medical trials, fish-oil supplements supplying at least 3 gm a day of omega-3 brought about real, if modest, reductions in the number of tender joints and amount of morning stiffness, as well as allowing many of the test subjects to cut down on their pain medication.

Q. Is there an omega connection to asthma?

A. Asthma definitely has a fatty-acid connection— a glut of omega-6. Omega-6 supplies the villainous eicosanoids, which not only induce bronchospasm (constricting of the bronchial tubes, which closes down the air supply), but make breathing even chancier by causing the air passages to swell and fill with mucous. It's not surprising that deaths from asthma have shot up in recent years. Children are especially vulnerable.

Scientists have known about the omega-6 eicosanoids and asthma for a while, but didn't make the connection with the big dietary change of the past thirty to forty years. Dr. Harumi Okuyama and his colleagues from the medical faculty of Nagoya City University set the research world on its ear by showing that the rise of asthma in Japan was directly related to Japan's huge postwar increase in the consumption of omega-6 oils. Even if you eat fish once or twice a week, you may not be able to curb the eicosanoids that can flood your system if you take in, typically, ten to thirty times more omega-6 than omega-3. Supplements are almost a necessity.

K. Shane Broughton, Ph.D., and his colleagues at the University of Wyoming at Laramie found that fish-oil supplements eased bronchial distress in many, but not all, of their asthmatic subjects. Their study was based on the fact that asthma incidence is low in certain populations who eat a lot of oily fish. In their own subjects, those who responded the best to fish oil showed lowered amounts of pro-inflammatory leukotrienes, the omega-6 eicosanoids that are the recognized culprits in asthma. Omega-3s in fish oil are important for inhibiting overproduction of these nasty eicosanoids. Dr. Broughton suggests that one reason fish oil doesn't always relieve bronchial symptoms might be that some asthmatics' intake of omega-6 oils is so high, it suppresses any beneficial actions by the omega-3s.

Q. What about allergies?

A. Dr. Okuyama says that allergies are part of the same picture. They've risen enormously in Japan, too—about one-third of Japanese babies now show allergic symptoms, including allergic dermatitis and food allergies. Many allergic reactions are tied to a surge in pro-inflammatory omega-6 eicosanoids. In Dr. Rudin's pilot study, a number of patients displayed an easing of allergies after switching from omega-6 oils and margarines to flaxseed oil or fish oil.

Allergies and asthma are too complex for simple answers, but if you're concerned about either ailment, a logical, safe first step would be to increase your omega-3 intake while at the same time cutting back drastically on omega-6 oils, trans-fatty acids, stick (firm) margarines, and all packaged foods containing them. You'll learn how to do this in Chapter 5.

Q. Can the omega-3s help my immune system?

A. If a splinter in your finger causes an infection, the swelling, heat, and tenderness you feel are created by white blood cells and other "soldiers" of your immune system engulfing and destroying the bacteria before they can spread to other parts of your body. Inflammation is normal to the healing process. However, sometimes, an inflammation can become more of a problem than a cure—for example, when the white blood cells remain active long after the original problem has resolved or when the immune system overreacts to a relatively harmless substance such as ragweed pollen or cat dander. We now know that the omega-3 fatty acids can rein in an immune system that is reeling out of control.

You may not need just a stronger immune system, but a "smarter" one. According to Dr. Simopoulos "a hyperactive or misguided immune system, not a sluggish one," is behind many health problems. A "smart" defense system, she says, "knows when to attack, what to attack, and when to hold back."

When your diet is too high in the omega-6 oils, Dr. Simopoulos explains, "your body speeds up production of a number of substances that can cause fever, pain, irritation, and swelling." For example, inflammations that persist often involve leukotriene B_4 (LTB$_4$), a powerful recruiter of white blood cells. Luckily, the omega-3s can inhibit excess production of LTB$_4$. The omega-3s can also curb the overproduction of a signaling protein called interleukin-1, which in normal amounts is part of a well-functioning immune system. Tests show that omega-3 fish-oil supplements cause big reductions of interleukin-1, both in humans and in lab mice.

Q. What are some immune diseases that can be helped by the omega-3s?

A. One man in Dr. Rudin's pilot study had suffered for two years with a hair-follicle inflammation in his nose that didn't respond to standard antibiotic and steroid treatments. The condition cleared up fully after the man took flaxseed oil for six weeks. While two women in the study who were severely crippled from rheumatoid arthritis didn't improve, two others who had had the disease for years but were not crippled showed almost complete remission beginning two months after the start of the study.

Another patient entered the study after five years of suffering with discoid lupus, an immune disorder thought to be related to lupus that causes reddened, damaging lesions to form on the face and upper body. This patient, according to Dr. Rudin, "began to show improvement two weeks after starting the flaxseed-oil regimen, as his dry, leathery hands softened. By two months, his hands were reasonably normal, and the painful cracking had disappeared. . . . Most impressive was a growth of firmly rooted hair on the 40 percent of the scalp that had not been irreversibly scarred.

"That the flaxseed oil caused the improvements was very clear," Dr. Rudin says. "When the patient stopped taking the oil for only two weeks, his skin began to dry and his facial lesions returned. The situation improved again when he resumed the oil supplements."

Dr. Rudin also saw improvement in a number of cases of seborrheic dermatitis, a skin condition that's characterized by flaking, red, patchy eczema around the hairline, eyebrows, nose, and cheeks.

Q. What about lupus and other immune disorders?

A. A series of recent medical trials demonstrated clear benefits from omega-3 fish oils in a very serious immune disorder, lupus (systemic lupus erythematosis). In addition, a number of studies have shown that persons suffering from chronic inflammatory bowel diseases—specifically, ulcerative colitis or Crohn's disease—respond to fish-oil supplements, which help ease the symptoms and reduce the need for the usual medications. In healed bowel tissues, the population of pro-inflammatory omega-6 leukotrienes has been shown to be markedly reduced.

A kidney disease known as immunoglobulin A (IgA) nephropathy has enough persistent inflammatory aspects to be classified as an immune disorder. Until recently, there was no safe, effective treatment to slow down the progression to renal failure in the most serious cases. Fortunately, in trials using fish-oil supplements, there were enough encouraging improvements in patients to warrant two major studies—one of them by Mayo Clinic doctors—in which the results of the use of fish oils alone, or of the use of fish oils compared with the use of steroids, are being evaluated over a two-year period.

Q. I heard that the omega-3s are good for the eyes. Is that true?

A. The omega-3s are not just good for the eyes, but indispensable. The retina of your eye needs lots of the most polyunsaturated omega-3 of all—DHA. The fluid quality that DHA imparts to the membranes enables your retina to convert with lightning speed the images it receives into electrical signals to be sent to your brain. Using its own DHA-rich neurons, the brain then lets you know what you're seeing. In one study, baby monkeys on a DHA-deficient diet lost some keenness in their vision and had slower-than-normal responses to visual signals. Premature human babies on either breast milk, which normally supplies DHA, or DHA-fortified formula can process visual images faster than babies on standard American formulas, which do not yet contain DHA.

Q. What about glaucoma and macular degeneration? Can the omega-3s help them?

A. Glaucoma, the ailment in which high fluid pressure within the eye damages the optic nerve, has diverse causes, but many are related to vascular problems. For example, persons more likely to get glaucoma are those who suffer from high blood pressure, heart disease, increased blood viscosity ("sludgy" blood), and/or poor circulation in the carotid arteries that feed the ocular areas. Enough research has accumulated just in the last ten years to verify that the omega-3s are a natural aid in preventing or correcting these blood-vessel disorders.

It's long been recognized that cigarette smoking increases a person's chances of developing glaucoma. One reason is that the internal diameter of the blood vessels actually narrows after a person smokes. By constricting the blood vessels, nicotine reduces the circulation to the retina. Now, the results of two long-term studies, involving more than 50,000 nurses and physicians, have proven that the chances of developing another serious eye disease that can lead to blindness—macular degeneration—will skyrocket if you smoke a pack or more of cigarettes a day. The macula, in the center of the retina, makes it possible for you to do such things as read, see straight ahead, and focus on fine details. Drs. Ronald Klein and Barbara Klein of the University of Wisconsin Medical School note in the *Journal of the American Medical Association* that smoking may damage the arteries in the macula the same way it's known to damage the coronary arteries. Smoking not only undermines the effectiveness of the protective antioxidant nutrients, they suggest, but might increase the stickiness of the blood cells responsible for clotting as well as reduce HDL levels. Again, omega-3 fatty acids in the diet along with plentiful antioxidant nutrients are now recognized to be a first line of defense against just this kind of assault on your circulatory system.

Q. Do the omega-3s have any effects on dyslexia?

A. At the University of Survey, England, daily doses of 480 mg of DHA for one month significantly improved the "dark adaptation" (night vision) of all five adults dyslexics participating in research trials. Starting in childhood, dyslexics have lifelong problems with reading in spite of having normal vision and intelligence. A brain defect processing and interpreting printed words and letters is one suggested explanation. The researcher Professor B. Jacqueline Stordy also observed in informal studies that DHA supplements improved reading ability and behavior in dyslexics. In general, many more males than females are dyslexic and also suffer disproportionately from ADHD. Do you suppose it's only a coincidence that infant boys also have higher omega-3 requirements than infant girls?

So, how doable is a daily intake of 480 mg of DHA? Very. About ½ C of either trout, salmon, shark, tuna, herring, sardines, or mackerel provides about twice that much DHA. You can also buy DHA supplements at health food stores and pharmacies.

Q. Can the omega-3 oils help to ease common "female problems"?

A. One of these problems, premenstrual syndrome

(PMS), is the term used for a whole bagful of discomforts that peak just before the menstrual period starts. Although its causes are complex, PMS is eased by a balanced omega intake, which can soothe away nervous tension and anxiety. At a cellular level, the omega-3s keep in check any omega-6 eicosanoids that might otherwise set off little "prairie fires" of irritation and inflammation at this vulnerable time of a woman's cycle.

Menstrual cramping should be mild and barely noticeable, but sometimes menstrual pain (dysmenorrhea) can be so severe that it forces young girls and women to take to their beds or to live on aspirin or similar drugs. Painful cramps are caused by overly strong contractions of the uterus in response to a certain prostaglandin derived from dietary omega-6 AA. (In fact, in normal childbirth, a huge surge of this prostaglandin signals the beginning of labor.)

Women who eat fish regularly are much less apt to have painful periods. This is logical because the omega-3 oils in fish keep too many of the critical prostaglandins from being churned out. In two months of treatment of forty-eight adolescent girls who tended to have severe menstrual cramps, the girls who took small (1.8 gm) daily doses of EPA and DHA from fish oil had much less pain than the girls given placebo pills.

Q. The omega-3s can make life easier for women of childbearing age, but what about women going through menopause?

A. Dwindling female hormones after menopause can cause thinning of the vaginal tissues and diminished lubrication. This may lead to vaginal dryness, itching, irritation, and pain during intercourse. Dr. Rudin writes, "Inadequate vaginal lubrication may be avoidable, to a large extent, when the body's omega-oil balance is right. All bodily secretions depend on how well each secretory cell functions. Essential fatty acids provide the molecules needed to build healthy secretory cells, including those in the glands that lubricate and moisten vaginal tissues. Two of the women in my study reported an increase in vaginal secretions after a few months of flaxseed-oil supplements."

Menopausal depression can affect many women. One of Dr. Rudin's volunteers reported being a cheerful, lively person before menopause had begun eight years earlier, but became depressed and anxious, beset with weeping spells and the inability to think clearly. When treated with estrogen, her mood had improved, but she developed tender, lumpy breasts. When her doctor stopped the estrogen, her scary breast symptoms cleared, but her low spirits returned. At this point, she volunteered for the pilot study. After a few months, the flaxseed-oil regimen enabled her to stop taking the hormone pills. Dr. Rudin writes, "Her mood vastly improved, and a number of other uncomfortable symptoms—including severe hot flashes—diminished."

Q. Is it true that menopause is easier for the women in Japan than for western women, and is this related to omega-3 intake?

A. Today's spotlight on menopause has brought to the world's attention the scarcity of symptoms in the women in Japan, where there is no equivalent term for "hot flashes," since so few menopausal women experience them. Japanese doctors, unlike American ones, rarely prescribe hormone-replacement therapy. The traditional Japanese diet employing many soy foods such as soybeans, miso, tempeh, and tofu is thought to be a big reason for the smooth sailing at menopause. Soy foods supply lignan and plant estrogens (phytoestrogens) such as genistein, which act like weak estrogens. In the high amounts eaten, they appear to ease the symptoms caused by the lowered hormone levels at menopause.

In addition to soy foods, the centuries-old diet of Japan is based on hunting and gathering—from the sea. The traditional omega-6 to omega-3 intake ratio is 2.8 to 1. This undoubtedly gives the omega-3s a powerful role that may be just as vital as that of the phytoestrogens in making menopause a breeze. Japan's older women, unlike its young folks, still stick to the traditional foods. It's the young Japanese, who eat less fish and more commercial foods prepared with omega-6 oils, that are the driving force behind today's higher (5 to 1) omega-6 to omega-3 ratio. Maybe, when today's young women reach the age of menopause, Japan will coin a term for hot flashes after all.

Q. What about osteoporosis and fatty acids?

A. Osteoporosis can be helped by the omega-3s, too. Loss of bone density and fragile bones seriously reduce the quality of life for many women after menopause, and for elderly men as well. New research indicates that the fatty acids have key roles in bone remodeling, the process by which worn-out bone is replaced regularly by healthy new bone. Yes, your bones are actually living tissues.

Certain omega-6 eicosanoids have an opposite effect on bones. At low, or normal, concentrations in the blood, they stimulate new bone to form. When there is too much of these eicosanoids, however, they inhibit bone formation. This is where the omega-3s come in—they keep the omega-6-eicosanoid output at normal, non-trouble-making levels. Bruce A. Watkins, Ph.D., of Purdue University in Indiana, saw an increase in bone formation, plus improved mechanical properties of the bones, in lab animals when he reversed their high-omega-6, low-omega-3 diet.

Osteoclasts are the cells that break down, or resorb, bone; osteoblasts are the cells that build bone. When resorption outruns bone-building, osteoporosis results. Researchers suggest that the omega-3s help to dampen overzealous osteoclasts, which may be getting too many signals from an excess of omega-6 eicosanoids. The omega-3s may also fight osteoporosis by stepping up the activity of a hormone called insulinlike growth factor. Insulinlike growth factor encourages the growth and remodeling of bone, but its activity tends to dwindle in older men and women.

Dr. Watkins found that antioxidant nutrients, particularly vitamin E, also are needed to guard bone and cartilage tissue from inflammatory damage induced by too much omega-6 eicosanoids. He writes, "Future research on dietary lipids and antioxidant compounds in bone biology may complement the current hormonal therapy for osteoporosis."

5.

Using the Omega-3s

Adding the omega-3s to your diet is not a difficult thing to do. They're found in many delicious foods that are readily available in your local supermarket and health food store. In this chapter, we'll discuss what foods are good sources and how to add them to your diet. We'll also discuss how to balance your omega-3 to omega-6 intake, and how to improve your pet cat's and dog's diets, too.

Q. Okay, I agree I need more omega-3. What's the best way to balance my intake?

A. Most people will need to drastically reduce the amount of omega-6 they consume and greatly increase the amount of omega-3. The ideal ratio of omega-6 to omega-3 is in the range of 3 to 1, 2 to 1, or 1 to 1. Most people consume these fatty acids in ratios of 20 to 1 or 10 to 1. You can create a better ratio of dietary omega-6 to omega-3 by:

❑ Avoiding or limiting your consumption of salad dressings, margarines, and commercial baked goods such as breads, muffins, cakes, and donuts. Baked goods from traditional European-style bakeries cause less of a problem because they are made with butter instead of cooking oil.

❑ Limiting your intake of corn, safflower, sunflower, cottonseed, peanut, soybean, and sesame oils, all of which are high in omega-6 fatty acids.

❑ Reducing your intake of foods made with lightly or partially hydrogenated oils.

However, simply avoiding omega-6 and transfatty acids is not sufficient. You also have to increase your intake of omega-3 fatty acids. (Not increasing omega-3 is where most low- and zero-fat diets go wrong.) Start by using flaxseed oil, which provides about 2 gm of LNA and 1 gm of LA per teaspoon. Other good oils are perilla oil, available in Asian countries and Asian grocery stores, and hempseed oil. However, all of these oils can go rancid unless refrigerated, so keep them cool. Flaxseed oil should taste mellow; a bitter taste means it's rancid.

Some oils contain moderate amounts of omega-3, but much more omega-6. These oils include canola (rapeseed) oil, walnut oil, wheat germ oil, and soybean oil. Canola oil is high in omega-9 fatty acids, as is olive oil. The omega-9 fatty acids are healthy, and extra virgin olive oil is preferrable to canola oil, though more expensive.

Q. What foods are high in EPA and DHA?

A. These omega-3 fatty acids are found in all fish, since they help to insulate against the cold. The fish with the highest levels of EPA and DHA are herring, mackerel, salmon, sardines, trout, whitefish, striped bass, bluefish, and tuna. These foods provide about 1 gm or more of EPA, plus DHA, per 100 gm ($3\frac{1}{2}$ oz, or about $\frac{1}{2}$ C) of fish.

Other types of fish are modest sources of EPA and DHA. These include carp, catfish, cod, flounder, haddock, hake, halibut, mullet, perch, pike, pollock, and smelt. In addition, crab, lobster, shrimp, clams, mussels, octopus, oysters, scallops, and squid contain a little EPA and DHA.

Q. What about nonfish sources of the omega-3s?

A. Flaxseed is the richest nonfish source of LNA, which the body converts to EPA and DHA. A rounded tablespoon of milled flaxseed provides 2 gm of LNA and .5 gm of LA. Other natural but more modest sources of LNA (and some LA) are Brazil nuts, walnuts, butternuts, chia seeds, hickory nuts, macadamia nuts, roasted or cooked soybeans, soybean sprouts, beans (various types), peanuts, olives, spirulina, spinach, purslane, oat germ, wheat germ, lamb, pork, and some cheeses (Roquefort, cream cheese, and cheddar).

Q. Can I cook, bake, and fry with flaxseed oil?

A. Although there's some controversy about whether you should cook with flaxseed oil, the recorded use of flaxseed oil as a cooking oil goes as far back as nine thousand years in areas of the Near East. Soldiers of the Roman Empire marched with rations of bread baked with flaxseed. China, the third largest flax grower in the world, has used flaxseed as a food oil for at least five thousand years. Germany uses 66,000 tons of flaxseed a year in baked breads and buns. Recent studies show little or no loss of LNA when milled flaxseed is baked as an ingredient in muffins or bread. Cooking also doesn't cause LNA or other fatty acids to oxidize (break down). Baking and cooking seldom expose fats and oils to temperatures above the boiling point (212°F or 100°C).

One test showed that stir-frying with flaxseed oil seemed to be okay, but only if the oil temperature was kept below 300°F (149°C). At higher temperatures, a fishy odor was detected, and significant levels of oxidation products appeared. Many flax-oil enthusiasts prefer, however, just to use the oil in salad dressing and home-baked goods, and stirred into soup, cereal, and cooked vegetables. However, never deep-fry with flaxseed oil for health reasons.

Q. What oils can I use safely for sautéing and frying?

A. Natural (non-hydrogenated) animal fats, such as butter, poultry fat, and pork fats, as well as tropical fats and olive oil have been used in this way for thousands of years without bringing on epidemics of heart disease or cancer. Coconut, palm, and palm-kernel oils—the tropical fats—contain easily digested medium-chain fatty acids, which are more likely to be used up as fuel by your body than stored as fat. Since they're mostly saturated, all the above fats contribute very little to the pool of potentially harmful eicosanoids. ("Saturated" is not a dirty word. Your body makes saturated fats. Even breast milk contains more saturated fats than any other kind.)

Olive oil keeps coming up roses in study after study. Populations that depend on it have fewer life threatening "modern" diseases. It's very high in monounsaturated oleic acid, which doesn't turn into eicosanoids. Extra virgin olive oil is preferred by many researchers. Canola oil, too, is high in oleic acid, but it's also high in the omega-3s and omega-6s, which can turn into harmful products at high frying temperatures. (Make sure the canola-oil label does not say "lightly or partially hydrogenated," which translates into "trans-fatty acids.") Never use any fats or oils that you've already used for frying.

Q. I need more help with the amounts of the omega-3s I should be getting. Are there any guidelines I can follow?

A. For a clearer picture, let's talk first about grams of the omega-3 fatty acids. While the experts vary on the minimum amounts they recommend, they all agree on the safety of 4 to 8 gm of the omega-3s a day, with a minimum of 1 gm to be in the form of EPA plus DHA. Here are some easy ways to achieve this quota:

❑ $3\frac{1}{2}$ oz (about $\frac{1}{2}$ C) of salmon, sardines, herring, mackerel, trout, tuna, or whitefish, which supplies at least 1 gm of EPA plus DHA.

❑ 7 oz (1 C) of less fatty fish and shellfish, which supplies approximately 0.5 gm of EPA plus DHA.

❑ $3\frac{1}{2}$ oz of lamb (loin), which supplies 0.5 gm of LNA.

❏ 6 walnuts, which supply approximately 1 gm of LNA.

❏ 1 tsp of milled flaxseed, which supplies 0.7 gm of LNA.

❏ 1 C of cooked beans, which supplies approximately 0.7 gm of LNA.

❏ 3½ oz of roasted soybeans, which supplies 1.5 gm of LNA.

❏ 3½ oz of purslane, which supplies approximately 0.4 gm of LNA.

❏ 1 tsp of flaxseed oil, which supplies 2 gm of LNA.

❏ 1 tbsp of canola oil, which supplies 1.5 gm of LNA.

Q. What about my omega-6 requirements? How do I fulfill those without going overboard?

A. All of the above foods also contain omega-6 LA—yes, even fish has some. Just by having a small handful of fresh nuts and seeds—such as walnuts, sunflower seeds, Brazil nuts, peanuts, almonds, pumpkin seeds, sesame seeds, and macadamia nuts—every day, you'll get lots of omega-6 LA. It's almost impossible to avoid the omega-6s in a decent diet, and you shouldn't try to avoid it. In addition to all the "double-duty" foods and oils listed in the previous answer, you'll get omega-6 LA from corn, whole-grain cereals and breads, cheese, chicken, turkey, egg yolks, and liver. That's why adding gobs of omega-6 oils to salads and the frying pan upsets the balance we need for health.

Q. What's Better Butter?

A. If you love the taste of butter but the spread-ability of margarine, here's a simple way to get both. Melt 2 sticks of butter in a saucepan, then add between $\frac{2}{3}$ and $\frac{3}{4}$ C of your favorite oils (for example, flaxseed oil, olive oil, canola oil), singly or mixed. Stir well, pour into a container, cover, and refrigerate. The mixture will taste like butter but spread like margarine.

Q. How can I get milled flaxseed? What are the best ways to use it?

A. Flaxseeds themselves have their enthusiasts, but the nutrients are easier for you to absorb from the ground seeds. As of this writing, you can buy flaxseeds from health food stores and vitamin mail-order catalogs. In a small electric seed or coffee-bean grinder, quickly grind 3 to 4 tbsp of flaxseeds to a powdery meal, empty the meal into a little covered container or plastic bag, and refrigerate. Or, check the same sources for already-prepared milled flaxseed, also known as flaxmeal. As flaxseeds' popularity grows, so will their availability in regular markets.

Milled flaxseed can have a laxative effect, so start slowly with 1 tsp. You can stir it into juice, applesauce, yogurt, dry or cooked cereal, or soup. Many folks like to mix it with psyllium-husk powder and stir it into juice. Children benefit from it, too, but start them of with $\frac{1}{2}$ tsp. For adults, amounts of up to 3 tbsp are known to be safe, but can be too laxative for some.

Incidentally, neither flaxseeds nor flaxseed meal oxidize (go rancid) readily, since they contain antioxidants natural to all seeds. They actually have a long shelf life. However, refrigerate your milled flaxseed just as a precaution. Remember, flaxseeds are the best source of the cancer-fighting lignans— the blessing besides LNA that they bestow.

Q. What am I supposed to do if I or my family don't eat fish or shellfish?

A. You'll all have to eat lots more of the other foods that provide LNA. It's estimated you have to consume about ten LNA molecules before your body turns one of them into EPA.

Another possibility is to take fish-oil supplements. These supplements are available in health food stores and pharmacies, both in liquid form (which are easier for children to take) and capsules. Read the labels to be sure that adults and adolescents get at least 1 gm (1,000 mg) of EPA plus DHA from a day's supply. Young children may need less, depending on their ages. Still another choice is fairly new, but growing in popularity—vegetarian EPA or DHA supplements, made from marine algae.

It's especially important for pregnant and nursing mothers who don't eat seafood to supplement their diets with these higher-chain omega-3s. Studies show that nonfish-eating vegetarian mothers supply their nursing babies with very low levels of DHA in their breast milk.

Q. Should I take additional vitamin and mineral supplements with my extra omega-3s?

A. There's one admonition when consuming high amounts of the omega-3s: protect your newly refurbished cell membranes with antioxidant nutrients. A higher omega-3 content in membranes makes them more vulnerable to oxidation. Yes, even in

your body, oxidation can happen, not too different-
ly from the way oils go rancid.

Vitamins A, C, and E are major protectors of your
lipid membranes. Make sure your daily multivitamin supplement provides at least 5,000 IU of A, 500
mg of C, and 100 mg of E. Even conservative physicians often recommend a daily multivitamin pill
that has at least 100 mg of E; many studies attest to
long-term safety of 400 to 800 mg daily.

A protective amount of the trace mineral selenium—200 micrograms daily—can be gotten from
supplements and/or selenium-rich foods such as
fish, shellfish, and liver.

Additional antioxidant help comes from a very
large group of compounds in fruits and vegetables called carotenoids. These compounds include
alpha- and beta-carotene, lutein, zeaxanthin, and
lycopene. Apricots, sweet potatoes, and leafy greens
are good sources of beta-carotene. Carrots and
pumpkins supply both alpha- and beta-carotene.
Lutein and zeaxanthin are present in leafy greens
and red peppers. And lycopene is found in toma-
toes, tomato sauce, guava, and watermelon.

Polyphenols and bioflavonoids form another
huge group of plant-derived defenders. They're
contained in, among other foods, red grapes, pome-
granates, mangoes, citrus fruits, plums, cherries,
blueberries, blackberries, and green tea.

Also, many of these foods are good sources of vitamins C and E, so it makes sense to eat at least five servings of fruits and vegetables a day—or even seven, as recommended by Dr. Simopoulos.

Q. How about my dog and cat? Are omega-3s good for them, too?

A. It shouldn't surprise you that the omega-3s are important for pets, too, since much of what we know about the omega-3s comes from animal studies. But here's a dismal twist on the pet-food story. The big push to beef up people's polyunsaturate intake was reflected in the pet-food industry. Most dog food is now made with grains, animal byproducts, and corn oil, which provide mostly omega-6 and hardly any omega-3 oils. Sound familiar?

The need for omega-3 was overlooked even for laboratory rats. Finally, in 1993, new official diet standards for these critters set by the American Institute of Nutrition called for switching from corn oil to soybean oil because corn oil "does not provide sufficient linolenic acid to meet requirements."

Whether the new standards for lab animals are affecting the whole pet-food industry is anyone's guess. Dog-food containers don't yet list omega-3 and omega-6 fatty-acid contents, but many commercial dog foods may still be too high in omega-6 and too low in omega-3. Hair loss; dull, dry coats; and skin disorders are some of the effects. In addition, an omega-3 deficiency in the mother can harm her unborn and, later, nursing pups at the times when the requirements are the highest for brain and retinal development.

If you're concerned for your dog, add a little milled flaxseed to his rations. Milled flaxseed is good for a dog's coat, helps to guard against arthritis and cancer, and stabilizes the immune system.

Cats are different. Imbalanced rations harm them because they require lots of omega-3 as preformed EPA and DHA, normally found in organ meats and fish. Felines have a harder time than dogs and humans in transforming LNA into EPA and DHA. Rats and mice may be the best at this and, therefore, may not be the best animal model for determining dog, cat, or human requirements.

Q. Can't the food industry find ways to get more omega-3 into our everyday foods to make it easier for us to stay healthy?

A. You'll be happy to know there is a big push in this direction, and it's gaining momentum every day. In 1997, the *British Journal of Nutrition* described a study by J.A. Lovegrove and coworkers, who examined whether processed foods enriched with EPA and DHA could make it easier for people to increase these in their diet. The enriched foods were breads, biscuits, cake, ice cream, orange drink, milk-shakes, low-fat spread, pasta, mayonnaise, vinaigrette, and milk-shake powder. The results? Not only did the volunteers find these foods entirely palatable, but after only twenty-two days of eating the enriched foods, their EPA and DHA blood-plasma levels had doubled.

More and more food providers in the United States, Canada, and Europe are competing to find practical ways to incorporate the omega-3s into their products while making sure the foods retain desirable tastes and textures. At the same time, poultry companies are beginning to sell eggs with yolks whose omega-3 content is many times higher than that of ordinary eggs. The omega-3 content of eggs goes up when the hen is given milled flax-seed, fishmeal, or microalgae. All of these developments are given every encouragement by scientists, whose goal is that farmers and animal breeders make a routine practice of giving high-omega-3 feed to livestock and farm-raised fish.

In essence, the food industry is being challenged to make the omega-3s as available to you today as they were to the hunter-gatherers who came before you. In the future, this will make it easier to maintain the correct omega-6 to omega-3 balance. Right now, you need to do this the hard way, by your own food and oil choices. Start today.

Conclusion

Not all fats are bad. In a modern world where most people consume far too much fat, and are simultaneously fat phobic, we've lost the ability to distinguish good fats from bad fats. And there is a big difference between them—a difference that affects our health.

Although many doctors point to the evils of saturated fats, found in beef and other animal foods, the greater problem is an imbalance of dietary fats. The modern highly refined and processed diet relies far too heavily on omega-6 fatty acids in salad dressings, baked goods, margarines, and other manufactured food products. These fats, while essential for health, increase the risk of inflammation, heart disease, cancer, and other disorders when we consume too much of them.

In contrast, the omega-3 fatty acids, also essential, tend to have the opposite effects, in large part because adding them to the diet helps to restore a more normal balance of dietary fats. You can restore omega-3 fatty acids to the diet by increasing your consumption of the omega-3s (by eating more fish or taking fish-oil capsules) and flax (by eating more milled flaxseed, flaxseed oil, or taking flaxseed-oil capsules). The first signs you'll likely notice are younger looking, healthier skin and fewer achy joints. But the benefits of the omega-3 fatty acids go far beyond, to reductions in your long-term risks for serious diseases. It's smart to rebalance your diet in favor of the omega-3s, and you will never regret doing so.

Glossary

Alpha-linolenic acid (LNA). Primary member of omega-3 family of essential fatty acids. The body converts LNA into eicosapentaenoic acid (EPA) or docosahexaenoic acid (DHA).

Arachidonic acid (AA). Member of omega-6 family of essential fatty acids. The body makes AA from the primary omega-6, linoleic acid.

Atherosclerosis. Buildup of fatty deposits, known as plaque, in arteries, causing narrowing of blood vessels.

Docosahexaenoic acid (DHA). Super-polyunsaturated member of omega-3 family, made from LNA. Found in high quantities in cold-water fish and marine mammals.

Eicosanoids. Natural hormone-like chemicals that regulate many body functions. Made by the body from omega-6 and omega-3 fatty acids.

Eicosapentaenoic acid (EPA). Member of omega-3 family of essential fatty acids. The body makes EPA from LNA. Found in high amounts in cold-water fish and marine mammals.

Leukotriene. One group of hormone-like chemicals—eicosanoids—made by the body from omega-6 and omega-3 fatty acids. Overproduction of leukotriene produced from arachidonic acid (AA) is associated with inflammatory disorders and bronchial spasms.

Lignan. A plant fiber that can form mammalian lignans in your body when acted upon by natural intestinal flora. Flaxseed is richest source. Known to have anti-tumor effects in humans. (Lignin, a different plant fiber related to cellulose, forms the woody cell walls of plants.)

Prostaglandins. Natural hormone-like chemicals—all made from omega-6 and omega-3 fatty acids—that regulate many body functions. Overproduction of those produced from arachidonic acid (AA) is associated with spasms in arteries, as well as inflammatory disorders.

Schizophrenia. A mental disorder often accompanied by hallucinations, "voices," delusionary thinking, and detachment from reality.

Thromboxane. An eicosanoid made from essential fatty acids. Overproduction of thromboxane made from arachidonic acid (AA) is associated with abnormal clotting in arteries.

References

Broughton KS, et al., "Reduced asthma symptoms with n-3 fatty acid ingestion are related to 5-series leukotriene production," *American Journal of Clinical Nutrition* 65 (1997):1011.

Cunnane SC, Thompson LU, eds., *Flaxseed in Human Nutrition* (Champaign, IL: AOCS Press, 1995).

Chen ZY, et al., "Stability of flaxseed during baking," *Proceedings of the 55th Flax Institute of the United States* (26–28 January 1994): 24–28.

Donadio JV Jr, "The role of omega-3 fatty acids in slowing progression of IgA nephropathy," *ISSFAL (International Society for the Study of Fatty Acids and Lipids) Newsletter* 4 (1997):7–10.

Hadley M, "Stability of flaxseed oil used in cooking/stir-frying," *Proceedings of the 56th Flax Institute of the United States* (20–22 March 1996):55–61.

Kang JX, Leaf A, "The cardiac antiarrhythmic effects of polyunsaturated fatty acids," *Lipids* 31 (1996):S-41.

Okuyama H, et al., "Dietary fatty acids—the n-6/n-3 balance and chronic elderly diseases," *Progress in Lipid Research* 35 (1997):409–457.

Pawlosky RJ, Salem N Jr, "Ethanol exposure causes a decrease in docosahexaenoic acid and an increase in docosapentaenoic acid in feline brains and retinas," *American Journal of Clinical Nutrition* 61 (1995): 1284.

Peet M, "Schizophrenia and omega-3 fatty acids," *ISSFAL (International Society for the Study of Fatty Acids and Lipids) Newsletter* 4 (1997):2–5.

Ratnayake WMN, et al., "Flaxseed: Chemical stability and nutritional properties," *Proceedings of the 54th Flax Institute of the United States* (30–31 January 1992): 37–47.

Robinson DR, et al., "Dietary marine lipids suppress continuous expression of interleukin-1-beta gene transcription," *Lipids* 31 (1996):S-23.

Rudin DO, "The major psychoses and neuroses as omega-3 essential fatty acid deficiency syndrome: Substrate pellagra," *Biological Psychiatry* 16 (1981):837.

Rudin DO, Felix C, *Omega-3 Oils: A Practical Guide* (Garden City Park, NY: Avery Publishing Group, 1996).

Rudin DO, Felix C, *The Omega-3 Phenomenon: The Nutritional Breakthrough of the '80s* (New York: Rawson Assoc., 1987).

Siguel E, MacKenzie A, "Distribution of w3 fatty acid levels and prevalence of low levels of w3 fatty acids in subjects participating in the Framingham Offspring Heart Study Cycle 4," in *Program and Abstract Book*, International Conference on Return of W-3 Fatty Acids Into the Food Supply, Bethesda, MD, 18–19 September 1997.

Simopoulos AP, Robinson J, *The Omega Plan: The Medically Proven Diet That Restores Your Body's Essential Nutritional Balance* (New York: Harper Collins, 1998).

Simopoulos AP, Salem N Jr, "Purslane: a terrestrial source of w-3 fatty acids," *New England Journal of Medicine* 31 (1986):833.

Stenson WF, et al., "Dietary supplementation with fish oil in ulcerative colitis," *Annals of Internal Medicine* 116 (1992):609.

Storlien LH, et al., "Skeletal muscle membrane lipids and insulin resistance," *Lipids* 31 (1996):S-261.

Thompson LU, et al., "Flaxseed and its lignan and oil components reduce mammary tumor growth at a late stage of carcinogenesis," *Carcinogenesis* 17 (1996):1373.

Uauy R, et al., "Rose of essential fatty acids in the function of the developing nervous system," *Lipids* 31 (1996):S-167.

Watkins BA, et al., "Importance of dietary fat in modulating PGE_2 responses and influence of vitamin E on bone morphometry," *World Review of Nutrition and Dietetics* 82 (1997):250–259.

Suggested Readings

Rudin D and Felix C. *Omega-3 Oils: A Practical Guide*. Garden City Park, NY: Avery Publishing Group, 1996.

Simopoulos AP and Robinson J. *The Omega Plan: The Medically Proven Diet That Restores Your Body's Essential Nutritional Balance*. New York: Harper Collins, 1998.

Index